QIGONG

SELF DISCOVERY &

HEALING

TECHNIQUES

UNLOCKING THE MYSTERIES OF QI

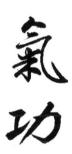

Raymond Wan
Tactical Health Coach

溫威文, 針療師

P.A.c., A.D.S., L.M.T., H.H.C.

Raymond has studied traditional Chinese acupuncture for 20 years and practiced Qi Gong for over 30 years. To gain better knowledge and understanding of the science of acupuncture; Raymond has continued to study medical acupuncture. In 2003, Raymond became a licensed medical massage therapist and also a certified holistic health counselor. In 2004, Raymond received his diplomat acupuncture practitioner certification, and after completion, he began teaching medical acupuncture. In 2005, Raymond became the director of a local medical acupuncture association; where he introduces and promotes medical acupuncture, while educating medical professionals and explaining the benefits of medical acupuncture to the public.

To further his knowledge of western medical treatment and US healthcare systems, Raymond continued his college education by focusing on human anatomy, physiology, disease developments, clinical nutrition, and clinical psychology. In 2011, Raymond received his Bachelor's Degree in Health Administration at University of Phoenix. In 2014, Raymond become certified Acupuncture Detoxification Specialist (ADS) from the National Acupuncture Detoxification Association (NADA). He specialized on using a technique called, "five needle ears acupuncture" which is used primarily to quit addictions. This technique is also used for weight loss, detoxification, and overall behavioral health (ADD, ADHD, Stress, Anxiety, Depression, etc.). To provide better treatment for his clients, Raymond loves to learn new skills. Currently he is working on his Doctor of Naturopathy in Original Medicine at The International Institute of Original Medicine.

QIGONG
SELF DISCOVERY &
HEALING
TECHNIQUES

UNLOCKING THE MYSTERIES OF QI

QIGONG SELF DISCOVERY & HEALING TECHNIQUES
UNLOCKING THE MYSTERIES OF QI
Published by The ME Marketing Group – 2016

ISBN: 978-0-9904933-5-8
Author: Raymond Wan
Cover design: Cover Creators
Copyright © 2016 Raymond Wan
First Edition in English

For further information, contact me at the following e-mail:
altcaresolution@gmail.com

Also be sure to visit my website at:
www.altcaresolution.com

Table of Contents

8th Movement: Holding the Sky

9th Movement: Pushing the Wall

10th Movement: Circling the Dan Dien

11th Movement: Circling the Middle Dan Dien

12th Movement: Holding the Sun and the Moon

13th Movement: Around the World and Back

14th Movement: Rise To the Middle Earth and Out

15th Movement: Going Out Of the Gate

16th Movement: Circle Around the Universe

17th Movement: Back to the Beginning Position

This is the End of the Movements

What is Qi?

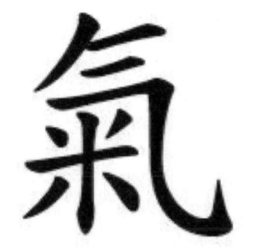

Common Translations of Qi

- Life Force

- Vital Energy

- Universe Energy

- Cosmic Energy

- Flow of Energy

- Spiritual Energy

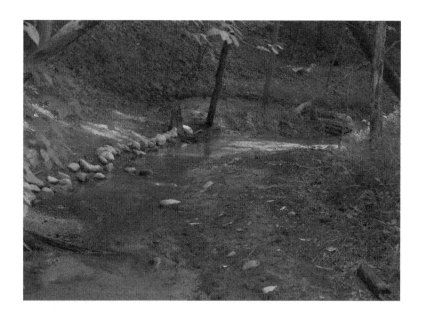

The Concept of Qi
Is Not Just in Chinese!!

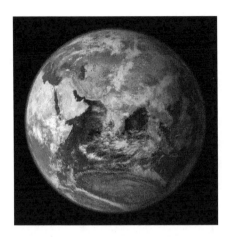

- Japanese – Ki

- Korean – Qi

- Vietnamese – Khi

- Hindu (yogic) – Prana

- Hawaiian – Mana

- Western - Energeia

Definition of Qi in

Chinese – English Dictionary

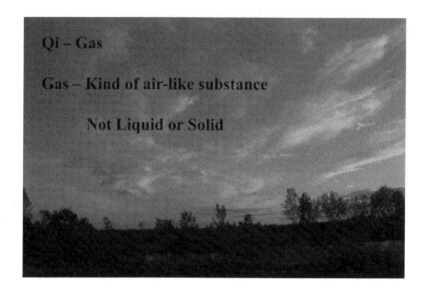

Qi – Gas

Gas – Kind of air-like substance

Not Liquid or Solid

<u>Chinese Characters</u>

- Qi – Mandarin

- Chi – Cantonese

In Chinese, it's pronounced   "Chee"

The Chinese Character of Qi

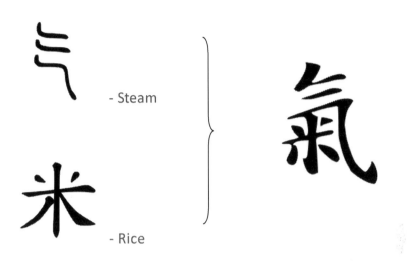

- Steam

- Rice

Meaning of the "steam rising" from Rice

Transformation of Energy from one from to other!

Traditional Chinese Belief Qi

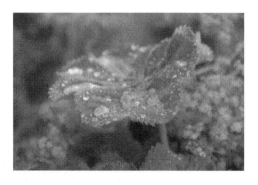

Qi is:

- Something we cannot see
- Supports our Life
- Destroys our Life

Examples:

Supports Our Life

Oxygen – We cannot live without oxygen

- We cannot see the oxygen but it supports our life

Destroys Our Life

Natural Gas – If we inhaled it we can die

- We cannot see it or smell it but if we inhaled it, it can kill us

Qi - an Overused Character

The Chinese use this character for everything

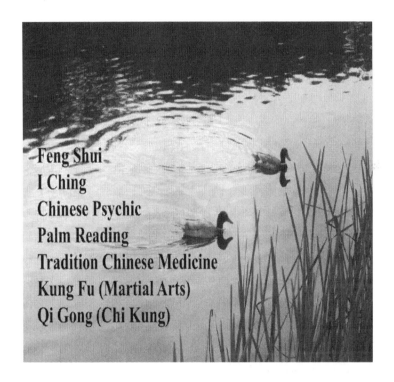

Feng Shui
I Ching
Chinese Psychic
Palm Reading
Tradition Chinese Medicine
Kung Fu (Martial Arts)
Qi Gong (Chi Kung)

Examples:

Chinese believe all is affected by a Qi

But Why?

Because…………………

Qi is a Complicated System

We can break it down into two categories

- Internal Qi

- External Qi

But they are also interchangeable

External Qi

- ◉ Belief that this Qi is outside our body

- ◉ It is our environment that could affect us

Examples:

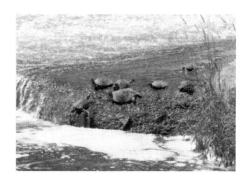

- Feng Shui

- Chinese Psychic

- Palm Reading

- I Ching

Use: Five Elements Theory & Yin-Yang theory

Believe outside environment: Space, Color, Shape, and Physical Location will affect the flow of Qi.

External Qi

External Qi Comes From.....

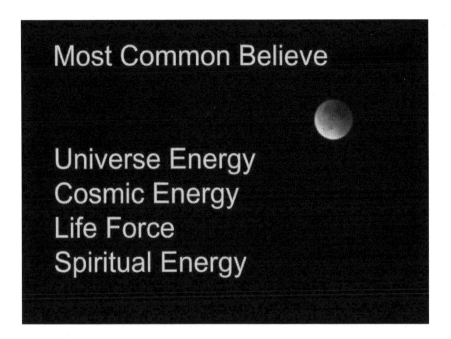

Most Common Believe

Universe Energy
Cosmic Energy
Life Force
Spiritual Energy

It Can Affect.......

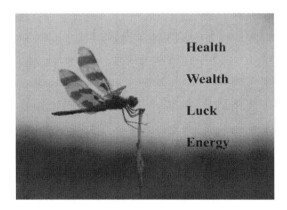

Health

Wealth

Luck

Energy

Internal Qi

Key Examples of Internal Qi

❖Traditional Chinese Medicine

❖Qigong or Chi Kung

❖Kung Fu (Martial Arts)

Where does this internal Qi come from?

◉ Element that we inherited from our parents

(Our Genetic Makeup it's in our DNA)

◉ Air we breathe

(Our Environment)

◉ Food we eat

(Transformation of energy)

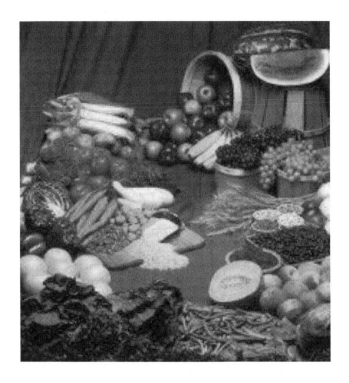

What Does That Mean?

Elements are inherited from our parents.............

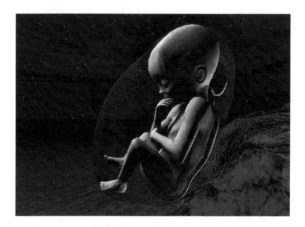

That means

- If your parents have a good Qi, you will be born with stronger Qi

- If your parents have bad Qi, you will born with weaker Qi

OMG!!!

Does that mean, if my family has history of:

- Diabetes

- Cancer

- Heart disease

- Stroke

- Any other genetic disease

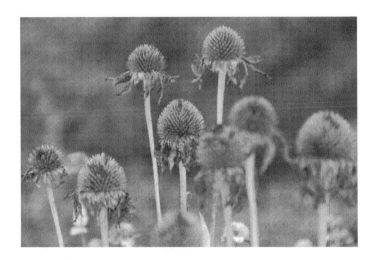

I will have it too??

NO!!

Three Different Sources of Qi

So far we have covered only one source of Qi:

- The element that we inherited from our parents

- (Our Genetic Makeup or In our DNA)

- But that is not the most important source of Qi

- Other factor can change our health outcome

Elements inherited from our parents

- The Qi that we are born with

    - This Qi storage is in our lower tan tien (or Dan Dien)

    - Also called (navel chakra, or Chi Hai)

- Chi Hal or CV6 acupuncture point

- Chi – energy

- Hai – Ocean

In other words, that is the ocean of Qi

Lower Dan Dien

- One thumb width below the navel

- All of our life force (Qi)

- ◉ That we born with storage in this point

- ◉ Every day we use up a little

- ◉ So we will grow older everyday

- ◉ Once it is used up………We Die!

Other Two Sources of Qi

- Air we breathe

(Our Environment)

- Food we eat

(Transformation of energy)

Our Living Environment

- If you live in a clean environment such as one with good sunlight, unlimited clean air and water, able to exercise every day, and have a good night sleep, you will live longer and healthier

- If you live in a toxic environment such as next to a factory that producing air pollution, a noisy environment, and/or living in the area don't have access to clean water, lack of motivation to exercise, and not able to sleep, you might develop many illnesses and it will be easier to get sick.

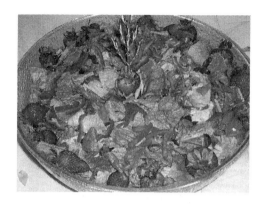

We Need Food

- Transforms to the energy we need, so we can get our work done

- Give us the nutrient we need to grow and heal our body

<u>Foods</u>

Clean foods such as GMO free organic vegetable and meat provides us abundance of nutrients, so our body can produce clean energy. (Or Clean Qi).

Unclean foods such as fast food and processed food, lack of nutritional value and it creates toxic effects in our body.

Our liver has to work harder to get rid of the toxins before we can absorb the nutrients, it wastes more energy to break it down before we can use it, and it weakens our whole immune system.

**We can talk more about
Food, Nutrition, and Diet
at other time!!**

Understand the Three Source of Qi

- The first one is "Element that we inherited from our parents" (Our Genetic Makeup or In our DNA)

- The second is "Air we breathe" (Our Environment)

- The third is "Food we eat" (Transformation of energy)

The first one is important factor of health but the second and third element can change the overall health outcome.

Example

Mary's parents are smokers and love to drink; her father also was diabetic.

When Mary was born, she might have had a weaker Qi. (Which made her easier to get sick?)

Her parents didn't change their lifestyle. It resulted in growing up with second hand smoke, fast food, processed foods, fried and sugary foods; her parents got drunk and fought most nights. (We can say she was living in a toxic environment.)

Mary always worries about become diabetic just like her father. (Added stress factor)

But one day she decided to change her lifestyle. She quit smoking, stopped eating processed and fast foods, added water in her diet, and start walking 15 minutes a day. After few weeks she started to feel lighter, and also lost a few pounds. The frequent headache and shortness of breath she experienced was gone.

Changing Your Health Outcome

Yes! Our genetic makeup is important, but the second and third factor can change the future of your health.

Qi is just like putting helium in the balloon, so the balloon can float in the air.

The first factor is the materials that created the balloon. Some may be better than the others.

After you put the helium in the balloon, every day afterward you can see the balloon getting smaller. (It's because the helium is lacking out)

Our bodies just like a balloon, and the materials that make up the balloon.

- If the quality of the materials is good, the balloon will take longer to deflate

- If the lower qualities of the materials are used, the balloon will deflate faster

Environmental Affect

- The second factor "Air we breathe" (Our Environment)

- The climate can affect the helium balloon

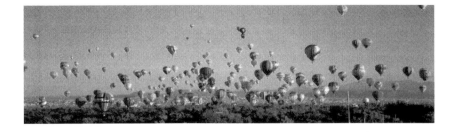

For example:

- In warmer climate the helium balloon might float longer in the air
- In cooler climate the helium balloon might not last as long

Food we eat

- The third factor "Transformation of energy"
- Very simple, if the helium in the balloon is leaking out little by little
- Then we can add a little helium back in the balloon every day
- Healthy eating can add the lost nutrients into the body
- Qigong practice just like add helium in the balloon.

Benefits of Qigong

- Increased or Decreased Circulation
  - Improve Circulation
- Bring more oxygen into the body
- Help blood to flow freely
- Decrease stress level
- Released toxins
- Increases the body's resistance to illness

- Strangling the whole immune systems

- And much more…………

Why we are Sick?

Well, in Chinese medicine

- Illness is cause by the blockages of Qi

- Stress level may cause blockages and the flow of Qi in the meridians

- Yin & Yang Qi out of balance

Traditional Chinese Medicine Beliefs

Our health depends on...................The balance of Yin & Yang Qi

Meridians

In Chinese medicine, Qi is transmitted through the twelve meridians. The Qi in the twelve meridians comes from twelve different organs: The heart, kidneys, gallbladder, lungs, stomach, spleen, liver, pericardium, bladder, large intestine, small intestine, and the triple heaters. These twelve meridians are located bilaterally in the body.

In the center of the body, are the governing vessel (GV) (Du Mai) and the consumption vessel (CV) (Ren Mai)

The Governing Vessels (GV) runs posterior of the spine, starting between the anus, and the tip of the coccyx, ending at the gum line of the two front teeth, and upper lip.

The Consumption Vessels (CV) runs through the anterior of the body, starting between the anus and near the major labia. It is located under the center of the tongue.

During Qigong practice, the goal is trying to conduct GV and CV.

To do so:

- Inhale and exhale through the nose.

- Close the mouth

- Tongue touches behind the two front teeth (This way it conducts the GV27 and CV24 at the endpoint)

    o The GV 27 and CV 24 are similar to the throat chakra.

- In the beginning of the session after you've cleared your mind, inhale and contract the anus, then exhale, and relax the anus. (This way it conducts the beginning points of the GV1 and CV1)

    o The GV1 and CV1 are similar to the root chakra.

One of the goals for Qigong practice is to allow the GV and CV to conduct naturally. This is what we call the fetus stage. The reason why is that, before a baby is born, since the lungs aren't developed yet, the fetus uses the diaphragm to breathe. The umbilical cord connects mother to baby, so that all the nutrients that the baby needs to grow, are provided by the mother.

 Therefore, the goal of Qigong practice is that we use our diaphragm to breathe, and to conduct our GV and CV, so that we can become centered and rooted back to the Mother Earth. (Or some people would say, "Connecting to the universe.")

Five Elements & Seven Emotions

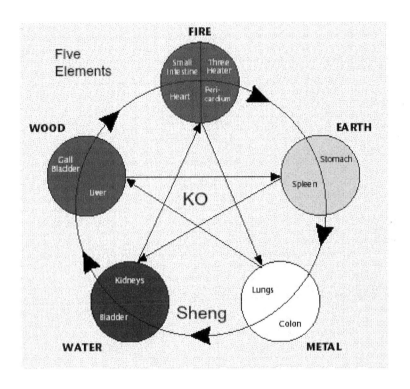

Five Elements

- The most complicated Chinese Medicine system

- Describe the relationships between Qi and the internal organs

- How our organs support and control each other's

- Maintain internal balance

Seven Emotions in the Chinese Medicine Theory

- Human emotions can affect the internal organs

- Our internal organs also can affect our emotions

Worry / Obsessed

- Linked to the Spleen

- Pensiveness or Over thinking

- Stagnation of Spleen Qi

- May cause:

  - Depression, anxiety, poor appetite, weakened limbs, abdominal bloating, menstrual irregularities, insomnia, constipation

Grief / Sadness

- Sadness is linked to the lungs

- Lead to respiratory problems, cause stagnation, bronchitis, asthmatic problems, chesty coughs

Grief

- Extreme grief (shock) is linked to the lungs

- Lungs Qi responsible for Qi circulation, shock affects the entire body

- May cause

  - Pallor, breathing problems, loss of appetite, constipation, urinary problems

Fear

- Linked to the Kidneys
- Excess will reverse the normal upward flow of kidney Qi
- May cause
  - Listlessness, lower back pains, urinary problems, desire of solitude, irregular menstruation

Anger

- Associated with Liver
- When too much Liver Qi rise (Liver Fire)
- May cause
  - Headaches, Flushed face, Dizziness, Red eyes

Joy

- Linked to the Heart
- "Inappropriateness" Negative aspect of Joy
- Can damage the lungs Qi
- The damage of the Heart Qi can lead to inability to concentrate
- May cause
  - Mental disorder, heart attack, stroke

The Yin Yang Theory

In Chinese medicine, Yin and Yang were in everything that existed.

In western medicine the human body is divided into different planes. In Chinese medicine, we use the Yin and Yang concept to divide the human body.

For example: The left side of the body is Yang. The right side of the body is Yin. Above the naval is Yang, below the Naval is Yin. The anterior part of the body is considered Yin, and the posterior of the body is Yang. But those energies are interchangeable.

For example: when we're sitting or inactive, we are considered to be in "Yin" condition. When we are moving our bodies will change to the "Yang" position. To maintain health, we must maintain the balance of Yin and Yang in our bodies.

Some people are born with more Yin energy, and some with more Yang energy.

To maintain health, we must maintain the Yin and Yang balance in our bodies.

Yin – Yang Concept

- ◉ Qi Created the Universe
- ◉ Yin & Yang created Qi
- ◉ Qi created Yin & Yang
- ◉ Yin & Yang are the greatest creation of Qi
- ◉ Qi is the mixer of Yin & Yang

- All living and non-living things are made-up of Qi

Confusing…..But Why??

The Origin of Qi

Long Before Time

- ◉ There was emptiness

- ◉ Two extreme opposite power flowing around

    - Pure Yin energy

    - Pure Yang energy

Some people call it:

- ◉ Pure good Qi

- ◉ Pure bad (evil) Qi

One Day

- ◉ This two pure opposite energy met and hit

- ◉ Because their equal power

- ◉ It created a rotation

- ◉ They were pushing and pulling each other

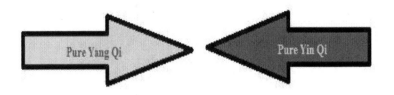

Yin & Yang were born!

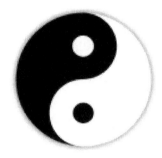

◉ Everything we see today is created by Qi

◉ Qi was created by the mixer of pure Yin & Yang Energy

◉ This mixer of pure Yin & Yang Qi created rotation

The rotation created

◉ Space & Time

◉ Day & Night

◉ Four Season

◉ Different dimensions

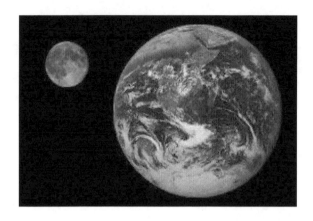

The Rotation of Yin & Yang cannot be stopped!

- This Yin & Yang Qi must stay in balance!

- If it stops or out of balance, the world and our universe will end

Is There Any Scientific Evidence??

Theory of Everything

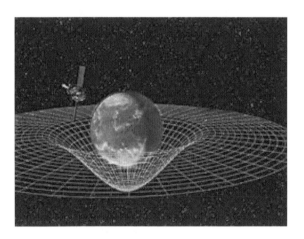

We might have to borrow few of the physical theories to find the answer

- String Theory

- Quantum Physics

- General Relativity

- Big Bang Theory

Big Bang Theory

- Long before time the universe was empty space

- Only had matter & anti-matter flowing around

- One day they collided and created a big bang

- Our Universe was born

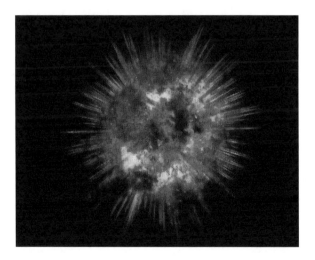

Quantum Physics

- Microscopic Particles (Atoms)

- Protons & Neutrons

- They are extremely small

- Extremely unstable

- They began pushing each other around in space

Atoms

- Everything is made-up of "Atoms"

- Each Atom contains a proton and neutron

- Protons carry a positive electron

- Neutrons carry a negative electron

- When Proton & Neutron get excited and mixed there electrons it created "Energy"

Gravity

- It is powerful but not that strong by itself.

- But it is heavy

- It pulling everything in

40

String Theory

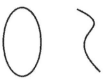

- Is the balance between

- Protons, Neutrons and Gravity

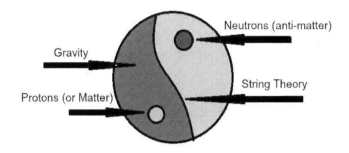

Traditional Chinese vs. Western Theory

Tradition Chinese Theory	Western Theory
Emptiness	Empty Space
Pure Yin Qi & Yang Qi	Matter & anti-matter
Two pure opposite energy meet and hit	Collided and created a big bang
Pushing & Pulling	Pushing & Pulling
Created rotation	Created rotation
Created space & time	Created space & time
Life was born All living & non-living things a mixer of Qi	Life was born Everything are make-up of Atom
Qi is mix of two opposite energy Yin Qi & Yang Qi	Atom is make up of Protons and Neutron, opposite energy

Does Qi Really Exist?

Scientific Research Showing

- Qigong master can change the electro frequency in their body

Use their hands to:

- Infrared electromagnetic waves
- Cause chemical changes in static water through mental concentration
- Ultraviolet absorption of nucleic acids
- Radioactive decay rates

Can Qi be measured in our body?

- The western medical scientist said Qi didn't exist
- But in 70's a group of Traditional Chinese Medicine doctor in China, invented an "Elector Acupuncture Scope", it can measure and locate the acupuncture points in the human body

New Discover in the 60's

- Dr. Robert O., Becker, discover electro activity is not limited in our nervous system
- He discovered that a crystal gel like substance are form in between the muscles
- It created a channel or pathway between our muscles
- This crystal gel like substance is highly conductive or resistant to electric currents

How does it Work??

- The neuron cells send and receive electro signals to our brain thrown nervous system

- But this pathway is not part of the nervous system

- This pathway is for sending signal for the body to heal

Water / Dehydration

- Water is one of the best conductors for electricity.

- Our body is made of 75% to 90% of water

- When the body is hydrated, this pathway become highly conductive electric currents

- When the body is dehydrated, this pathway become resistant to electric currents

- Physical injury can affect the function of this pathway

- Toxic buildup can also cause blockage in the pathway

<u>Food for Thought</u>

East vs. West

Traditional Chinese Medicine (EAST)	Western Science (WEST)
Qi is flowing in the 12 meridians (channels)	Electric currents are running through crystal gel pathway
The Qi in the meridian can be blocked.	This pathway can be highly conductive or resistant toward electric currents
illness is cause by the blockage of the meridian	Poor diet, Physical injury, internal toxic and dehydration can cause blockage
Qi can be measure by "Elector Acupuncture Scope"	The body's electricity can be measured
Qi	Electromagnetic Waves

How to get rid of the Blockage?

- ◉ Drink enough water

- ◉ Current water intake should be half your body weight change to ounce

Example: if you are 150 pounds

150/2 = 75, so you need 75 ounce of water daily

!

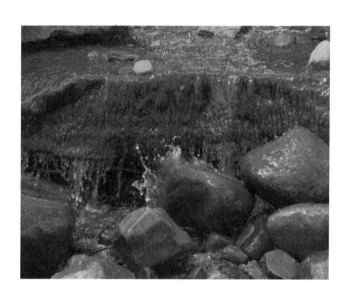

Chinese Theory

According to Huang Di Nei Jing, "The Yellow Emperor's Classic of Internal Medicine," one of the oldest complete medical textbook in the world that dates back over 4000 years old, written by Shen Nung who's the father of Chinese Medicine, wrote in detail describing how Qi affects the human body!

To Remove the Blockages

- ◉ Decrease Stress Level

- ◉ Diets

- ◉ Exercise

    - ○ (Kung Fu)

    - ○ (Qi Gong)

- ◉ Herbal Medicines

- ◉ TuiNa (Chinese Massage Technique)

- ◉ Maxbustion

- ◉ Acupuncture

How Many Kinds Of Qigong are Out There

There are many kinds of Qigong, but we can break it down to two major category

- Hard Qigong

- Soft Qigong

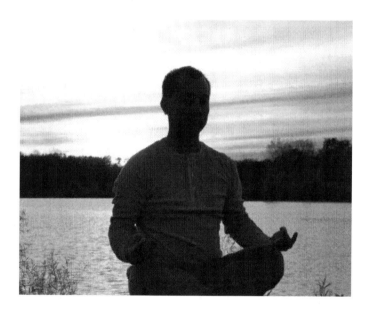

Hard Qigong

Commonly use in Martial Arts Training

The martial artist learns to:

◉ Change breathing pattern

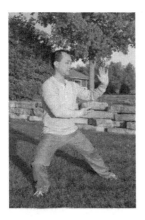

◉ Change mindset and ability to focus

◉ Increase their strength and power

◉ Ignore pain (During the fight)

This style of Qigong is internal Qi using externally.

Soft Qigong

- Internal Qi

- Self-Healing

- Heal others

There are many style of Healing Qigong

Different Style of Qigong

- Sound Qigong

- Laughing Qigong

- Walking Qigong

- Quiet Qigong or Sitting Qigong

- Movement Qigong

    - (Tai Chi) or (Yogi)

- Sexual Qigong

- Couple Qigong

Just to name a few.....................

What Style of Qigong Should I Learn?

- I am a lazy guy and don't like to move much

..........So, Sitting Qigong or Quite Qigong would be best for me

- If I was a very active person and could not sit still

- *Then Movement Qigong would work best*

- Married couples may like to improve their relationship or make it stronger

- *Couples Qigong would be the best*

What Kind of Qigong Will We Learn Here?

- ◉ Sitting qigong (For people able to sit on the floor Indian style)

    - ◉ Small Upper Body Movement

    - ◉ Chair qigong (For people unable to sit still on the floor)

    - ◉ Small Upper Body Movement

    - ◉ Laying down qigong (For people unable to sit still on the floor)

51

<u>Qigong practice</u>

- Re-discover ourselves

- Reduce or release our emotions

- Maintain balance

Before we start

- No food one hour before practice

- Wear loose comfortable clothing

  - Once you practice regularly, your body will start generate lots of heat

- A good comfortable sitting pillow

- This from is for people able to sit cross leg like Indian style for 50 minutes

  - Beginner might start with 5 to 15 minutes daily practice

3 Focal Points

1) Upper Dan Dien (Third Eye)(GV24.5)

   a. Pineal gland (master gland of all glands, it is our internal clock. It control all other glands)

   b. I call it the Switch

2) Middle Dan Dien (Heart Chakra)(CV17)

   a. Thymus gland (produce grown hormone for children, shrinks after the individual reaches maturity, but continues to stimulate the development of T cells, (disease-fighting white blood cells.)

   b. It is also our mental gravity point

   c. I call it the Sub-station

3) Lower Dan Dien (Navel Chakra)(CV6 Qi Hai)

   a. Life force storage point

   b. It is also our center gravity point.

   c. I call it the Car Battery or Bank

Breathing Techniques

- Use the Diaphragm

- Breathe with the diaphragm not the Lung

Disadvantages of Lung Breathing

- ◉ In normal day people breath with their lungs

- ◉ When we inhale, the rib cage have to move upwards to allow the lungs to expand

- ◉ To do so, the surrounding muscles most be contract

Causes

- ◉ Muscles tension

- ◉ Tension headache

During stress

- ◉ Weakling the lung function

- ◉ Add physical stress to the body

- ◉ Weakling the immune system

Benefit of Diaphragm Breathing

❖ When we inhale with our diaphragm, we can avoid neck and shoulders muscle engage

❖ Help reduce muscles tension especially the upper body, neck and shoulders

❖ Bring in more oxygen to your body

❖ Relax muscles

❖ Improve muscles flexibility

❖ Reduce tension headache

❖ Improve lung function

❖ Improve asthma

❖ Strengthening the immune system

How do I know I use the Diaphragm or Lung?

◉ Put your hand by your mouth

◉ Inhale with your nose then exhale with your mouth

◉ Bow the air to your palm and feel it

◉ Is it warm or cool?

◉ If it is warm, you used your lung

◉ If it is cool, you used your diaphragm

<u>Why and What Happens?</u>

- ◉ The air was warm because when inhales with the lung, all excess oxygen were warmed by the blood vessels in the lung. Therefore the exhaled air is warm!

- ◉ When you inhale with the diaphragm, the excess oxygen did not pass throw the lung. So the blood vessels did not warm up the oxygen when you exhale. Therefore the air is cool!

Now…You Get It!

Breath with the Diaphragm

- Slowly inhale, slowly exhale

- Focus on

- Upper Dan Dien

- Middle Dan Dien

- Lower Dan Dien

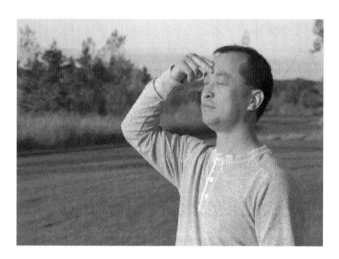

Beginner Qigong

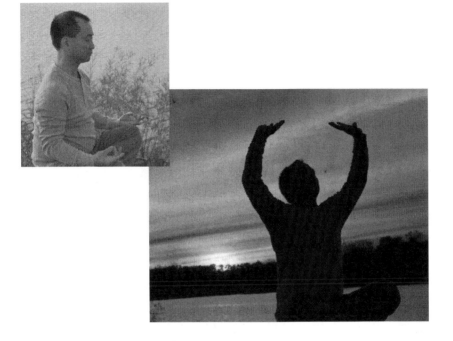

How to clear your mind

- Our human brain is like a 2 years old child, it never stop or able to stop.

- Therefore it is impossible to clear our mind.

- Instead let your brain or thought run wild

- We can give it a purpose or something to focus on

- The upper Dan Dien (Third Eye)

Focus on Upper Dan Dien

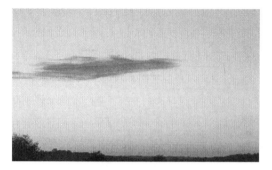

- Remember the upper Dan Dien is where the Pineal gland is at

    - The pineal gland is the master gland of all gland

    - It is our internal clock

    - It tells us when to sleep and when to rest

    - It controls all the other glands when to start working

- By focus on this point, we can manually reset our internal clock.

Here is How You Might Feel?

- After you close your eyes, you might see a white dot (some people see a black dot, some people see a colorful shadow) between your eyebrows (third eye). It doesn't matter what color or shape, just focus on that point.

- That dot may slowly disappear or expand, although it depends on the individual

- Your mind is clear now

If you still have a hard time to find your focus point, try to use a candle.

- ⊙ Light a candle put it in front of you

- ⊙ Look at the candlelight before you close your eyes

- ⊙ Now you should see a light between your eyes

- ⊙ Use that as your focus point

- ⊙ Relax and breathe

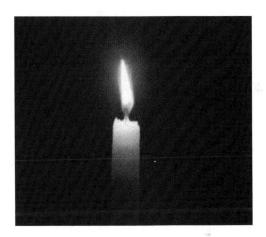

Beginning Position

- ⊙ Sit on pillow Indian style (Cross your legs)

- ⊙ Straighten your spine

- ⊙ Relax your shoulders

- ⊙ The tip of your thumb touching the tip of your middle finger

- ⊙ Relax your hands and rest them on your lap

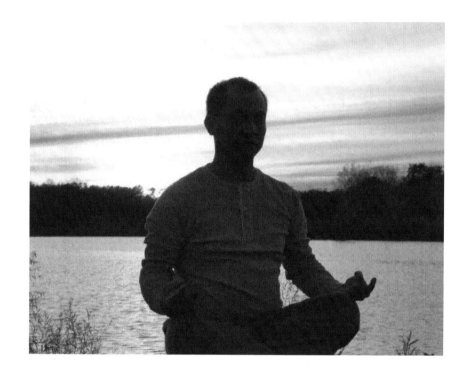

The Four Steps

First Step

Clear your mind

- Breathe with the Diaphragm

  - Slowly inhale, slowly exhale

  - Focus on Upper Dan Dien (Third Eye)

  - Every time when you exhale, let go of your emotions or thoughts

  - In each breath, the dot on your third eye appears smaller

  - Slowly inhale and exhale about 5 more times, your mind is clear

Second Step

- While exhaling, imagine this energy dot on your third eye slowly moving down to your middle Dan Dien

- Inhale focus on your middle Dan Dien.

- Then exhale, imagine this energy dot slowly moving down to your lower Dan Dien (center line, in front of the body)

- Inhale & exhale

- Using your Diaphragm

- Focus on the lower Dan Dien

- Spine straight

- Relax your shoulders

Third Step

- ◎ Focus on lower Dan Dien

- ◎ Inhale using your Diaphragm

  - When inhale using the diaphragm, it helps with putting the stomach and intestine downward

- ◎ Contract your anus

  - When contract the anus, it help putting the intestine upward

  - Remember when exhale, imagine this energy dot slowly moving down to your lower Dan Dien from the center line in front of your body

  - Combined movement created an internal massage

  - Imagine the beginning points of the GV and the CVs are conducting together and rooted to the ground, starting to share energy with mother earth.

Benefits

- relax the intestine

- Improve the strength and flexibility of the internal organs

- Remove toxic waste

- Improve bowel movement

- Reduce Headache

- Reduce fatigue

- Help for constipation

- Bloating

- Improve energy level

- Improve mental clarity

Step Four

- Exhale relax your anus

- Then inhale and Imagine this energy dot slowly moving Upwards

  - From the center of your spine in the back of your body

  - Moving upwards to the lower Dan Dien

  - Continue rising up to middle Dan Dien

  - Then moving up to the Bai Hui (GV20) or crown chakra (Imagine this point opening up, sharing the energy with the rest of the universe.)

  - Exhale – the energy from Bai Hui moving downward to the third eye

- We call this "Small Cycle"

- The goal is conducting the Governing vessel (GV) and the Conception vessel (CV) back to the fetus stage.

17 Movements

1st Movement-Holding a Pot of Soup

- After clear the mind and started the small cycle

- Next step inhale

- Slowly raise your arms up to the level of your heart (level to the middle Dan Dien) hold your arms in a circle.

- Relax your shoulders and elbows

- Palm facing inward

- Inhale and exhale with your diaphragm

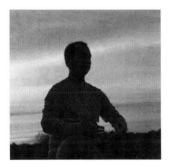

- Imagine the energy is circulating through your middle Dan Dien outward to your palms and fingertips.

- After you hold the position, you may begin to feel the energy filling the empty space between your arms and body.

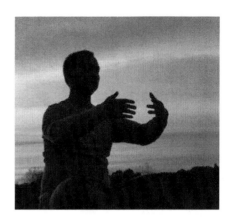

2nd Movement-Eating 3 Bowls of Soup

After the soup cooks for few minutes, it is time to eat

- ⊙ Exhale, slowly move your arms down to the level of your lap

- ⊙ Inhale, raise both palms upward and slowly move your arms upward along your body to the level of your nose

- ⊙ Exhale, both palm turn face down and slowly move downward along your body back to the lower Dan Dien

- ⊙ Turn palm face upward inhale, and repeat this breathing sequence 3 times

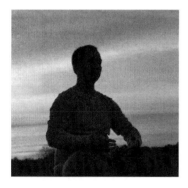

3rd Movement-Cooking Second pot of Soup

After inhale and exhale with the hand movement 3 times, you still hungry and need to cook more energy soup

- Slowly inhale and move the arms back up to the level of your middle Dan Dien

- Your palms face inward

- Relax your shoulders

- Relax your elbows

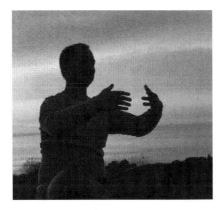

Imagine the energy is circulating through your middle Dan Dien outward to your palms and fingertips.

After you hold the position, you may begin to feel the energy filling the empty space between your arms and body.

4th Movement-Eating another bowl of Soup

- ⊙ After cooking the second pot of soup for few minutes, it is done and time to eat

- ⊙ Relax your shoulder and elbows

- ⊙ This time your palms face inward

- ⊙ Inhale, move your palms close to your nose

- ⊙ Turn your palms outward

- ⊙ Exhale, move your palms outward level to your middle Dan Dien

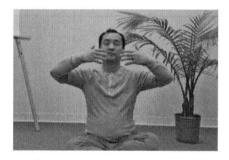

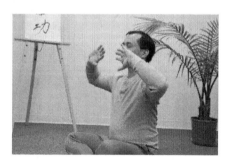

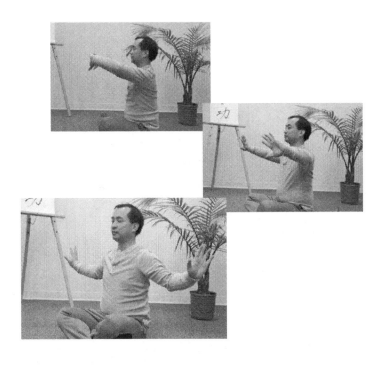

5th Movement-Too full, Share with everyone

- ◉ Inhale and relax

- ◉ Exhale, move your arms outward level to your shoulders

- ◉ Relax your shoulder and elbows

- ◉ Inhale and exhale

6th Movement-Pushing the Wall

- ◉ Your palms outward level to your middle Dan Dien

- ◉ Both hands move to the side of the body

- Finger point upward

- Elbow point downward and relax

- Move your middle finger backward (this opens up your acupuncture point "Lao Gong")

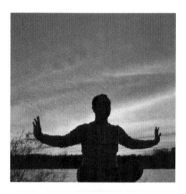

You should be able to feel the energy enter through the Lao Gong point, (P8) rushing down your arms to your middle Dan Dien, and down to the legs, all the way down to the bottom of your feet, at kidney 1 (Yong Quan or "Gushing Spring.") This encourages you to feel rooted to the ground and creates a stronger connection with mother earth.

7th Movement-Crossing to the Heavens

- Exhale, draw arms down,

- At the navel, start to inhale,

- Hands crossed at chest level,

- Continue to raise above the head

- Palms upward,

- Exhale, hold the position.

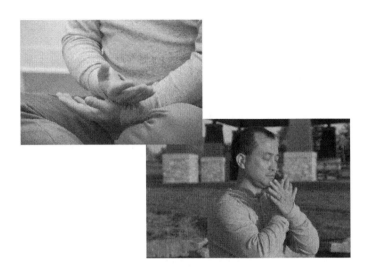

8th Movement-Holding the Sky

- ◉ Hold hands above the head, with palms facing upward

- ◉ Relax, continue breathing through the nose

- ◉ Continue for a few minutes

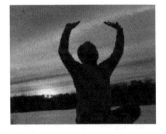

Imagine the energy starting to release through the center of your palms (P8). Feel the energy coming in through the GV 1 and CV 1 (The root chakra), just like a tree.

9th Movement- Pushing the Wall

- ⊙ From the position, "Holding the Sky,"

- ⊙ Exhale; draw both arms down slowly, to the level of the shoulders

- ⊙ Fingers pointed upwards with palms facing out

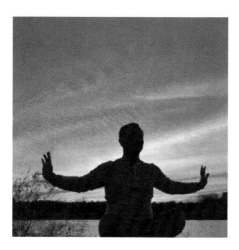

- ⊙ Pull the middle finger inward

- ⊙ Hold position for a few minutes

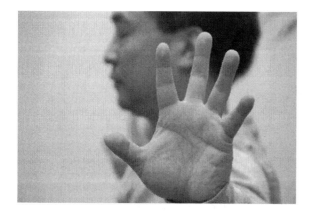

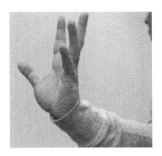

You should be able to feel the energy enter through the Lao Gong point, (P8) rushing down your arms to your middle Dan Dien, and down to the legs, all the way down to the bottom of your feet, at kidney 1 (Yong Quan or "Gushing Spring.") This encourages you to feel rooted to the ground and creates a stronger connection with mother earth.

10th Movement-Circling the Dan Dien

- After a few minutes exhale,

- Relax and draw the arms downward.

- Exhale, hand over hand, thumbs together in a circle and hold the lower Dan Dien.

- Relax and hold position for a few minutes

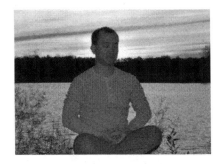

Your mind is focused. Draw all of your energy, and focus on the lower Dan Dien.

11th Movement-Circling the Middle Dan Dien

- ◉ After a few minutes slowly inhale,

- ◉ Raise your hands to middle Dan Dien, Maintain the fingers in a circular shape.

- ◉ Once you reach the middle Dan Dien, start to turn your wrist, palms facing downward.

Imagine the energy is slowly going up from the lower Dan Dien to the middle Dan Dien.

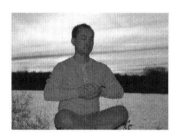
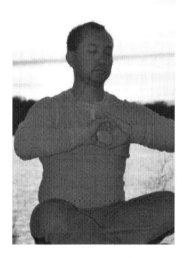

12th Movement-Holding the Sun and the Moon

- Continue inhaling

- Slowly open your hands

- Holding a circle with your thumb and index finger, slowly raise your arms up

- Raise hands over your head

- Look up, eyes focusing on the circle.

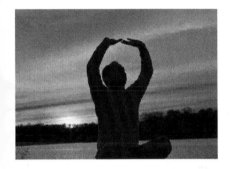 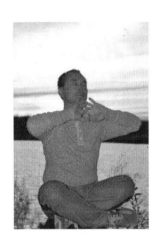

Feel the energy coming in from the center of your palm. (P8) In that instance, you should feel your third eye opening up. Feel the energy coming in through the circle to your third eye. This warm sensation should go all the way down to your lower Dan Dien, at the anterior of the body. Then coming back up through the posterior midline of the spine, up to the GV 20 (the crown chakra), and feel this point open up.

13th Movement-Around the World and Back

- ◉ After a few minutes

- ◉ Exhale

- ◉ Slowly move your arms all the way down to your lower Dan Dien

- ◉ Palm over palm facing upward

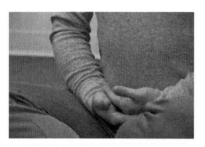

Guide all of the energy to the lower Dan Dien.

14th Movement-Rise to the Middle Earth and Out

- ◉ Inhale

- ◉ Raise your palms up to the middle Dan Dien

- ◉ Turn your palms outward, thumbs pointing down.

- ◉ Exhale

- ◉ Push the hands out

- ◉ Inhale

- ◉ Relax the elbows and shoulders

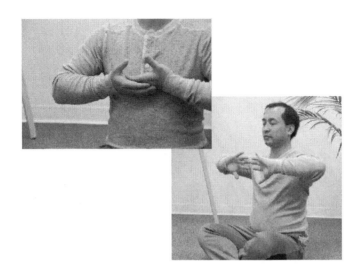

In this position, you should feel the Qi circling around your arms going out from your palms.

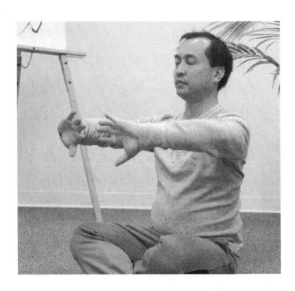

15th Movement-Going out of the Gate

- ⊙ Inhale

- ⊙ Move hands apart, fingers pointing upwards.

- ⊙ And then relax the arms (Hold position for few minutes)

- ⊙ Exhale drawing the arms down

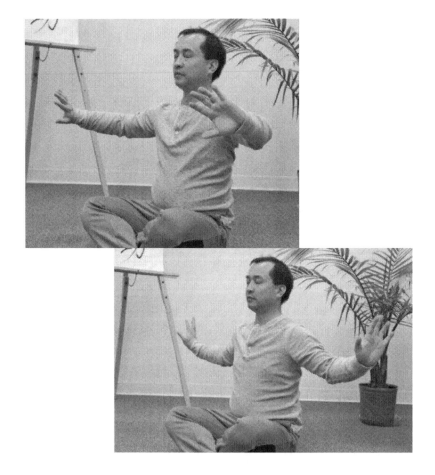

16th Movement-Circle around the Universe

- ◉ Inhale

- ◉ Raise palms up

- ◉ Hands crossing the chest over the head

- ◉ Exhale

- ◉ Draw the arms down slowly to the side of your body, and continue going down, hands going down to the lower Dan Dien, and slowly rising up

- ◉ Inhale

- ◉ Continue this movement three times

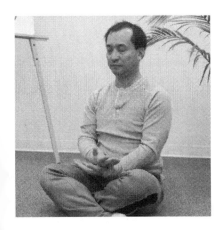

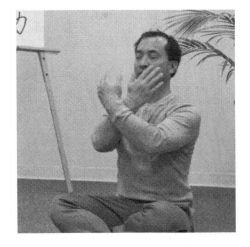

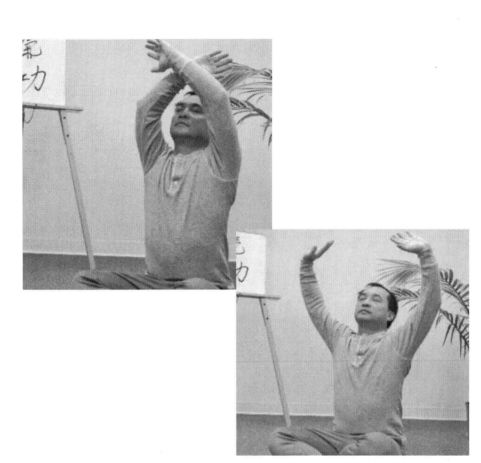

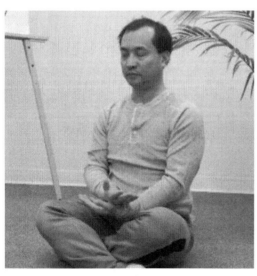

80

17th Movement-Back to the Beginning Position

- ◉ After the third circle move hands to the beginning position

- ◉ The tip of your thumb touch your middle finger

- ◉ Relax your hand and on your lap

Focus and guide all of the energy back to the lower Dan Dien.

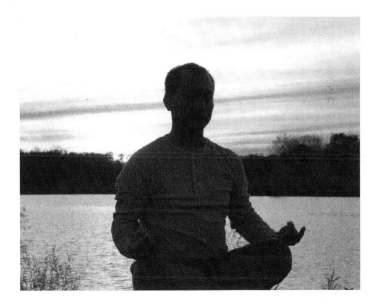

This is the end of the movements

- ⦿ Once you've guided all of your energy to the lower Dan Dien,

- ⦿ Take a deep, deep breath

- ⦿ Slowly open your eyes

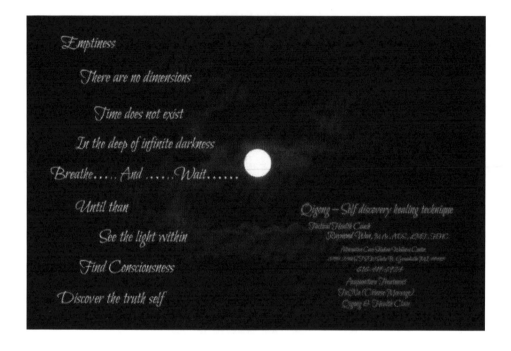

For further information, contact me at the following e-mail:
altcaresolution@gmail.com

Also be sure to visit my website at:
www.altcaresolution.com

39145520R00046

Made in the USA
Middletown, DE
15 March 2019